SURVIVING CERVICAL CANCER

NAVIGATING YOUR JOURNEY TO WELLNESS

JESSIE W. HARDISON

ISBN: 9798387408106

DEDICATION

This book is dedicated to my friend Catherine and to all those trying to get guidance on Cervical Cancer.

CONTENTS

INTRODUCTION

Cervical cancer is one of the most common types of cancer among women worldwide. It develops in the cells of the cervix, the lower part of the uterus that connects to the vagina. The disease is often caused by the human papillomavirus (HPV), a sexually transmitted infection, and it can be prevented by getting the HPV vaccine and regular cervical cancer screenings.

Despite the availability of preventative measures, many women are still diagnosed with cervical cancer every year. This diagnosis can be devastating, and it can be difficult to know where to turn for help and support. But the good news is that cervical cancer is often curable when detected and treated early.

In this book, we will provide a comprehensive guide to understanding cervical cancer, including its causes, symptoms, diagnosis, and treatment options. We will also address the challenges of living with cervical cancer and offer strategies for coping with the physical and emotional effects of the disease.

This book is written for women who have been diagnosed with cervical cancer, their families and loved ones, and anyone who wants to learn more about this disease. We hope that the information and guidance provided here will empower women to take control of their health and navigate the challenges of cervical cancer with strength, courage, and resilience.

OVERVIEW OF CERVICAL CANCER

Cervical cancer is a type of cancer that begins in the cervix, which is the lower part of the uterus that connects to the vagina. Survival rates for cervical cancer have improved significantly in recent years, thanks to advances in screening, diagnosis, and treatment.

The survival rate for cervical cancer depends on several factors, including the stage at which it is diagnosed, the size of the tumor, and whether the cancer has spread to other parts of the body. According to the American Cancer Society, the overall 5-year survival rate for cervical cancer is about 66%. This means that about 66% of women with cervical cancer are still alive five years after their diagnosis.

When cervical cancer is detected early, the survival rate is much higher. For women with localized cervical cancer (cancer that has not spread beyond the cervix), the 5-year survival rate is around 92%. However, it cancer has spread to nearby lymph nodes, the survival rate drops to around 56%.

Treatment for cervical cancer typically involves a combination of surgery, radiation therapy, and chemotherapy. The specific treatment plan will depend on the stage of the cancer and other individual factors. In some cases, a hysterectomy (surgical removal of the uterus) may be necessary to remove cancer.

After treatment, women with cervical cancer will need to be closely monitored for recurrence. Follow-up care may include regular physical exams, imaging tests, and Pap smears to check for abnormal cells in the cervix.

In addition to medical treatment, there are lifestyle changes that can help improve survival and overall health. These may include eating a healthy diet, getting regular exercise, and quitting smoking.

Overall, cervical cancer can be a serious and potentially life-threatening condition, early detection, and treatment can greatly improve the chances of survival. Regular cervical cancer screenings and prompt medical attention for any symptoms or abnormalities can help catch cancer early when it is most treatable.

Goals of The Book

Assuming that the book "Surviving Cervical Cancer" is a self-help or educational book aimed at those who have been diagnosed with cervical cancer or their loved ones, some possible goals of this book could include:

- To provide clear and accurate information about cervical cancer, including its causes, symptoms, diagnosis, and treatment options.
- To offer guidance and support for coping with the emotional and practical challenges of a cervical cancer diagnosis, such as fear, stress, and navigating the healthcare system.
- Provide a sense of hope and optimism.
- To educate readers about the importance of early detection and regular cervical cancer screening, and to provide information about ways to reduce the risk of developing cervical cancer in the future.
- To encourage readers to prioritize their health and well-being, and to provide practical advice on self-care and lifestyle changes that can help support recovery and prevent a recurrence.
- To address common misconceptions and stigmas surrounding cervical cancer, and to promote awareness and understanding of the disease.

Understanding Cervical Cancer

Cervical cancer is a type of cancer that develops in the cells of the cervix, which is the lower part of the uterus that connects to the vagina. It is the fourth most common cancer in women worldwide and can develop in women of any age, although it is most frequently diagnosed in women between the ages of 35 and 44.

The main cause of cervical cancer is the human papillomavirus (HPV), a sexually transmitted infection. HPV is very common and most women who are sexually active will have an HPV infection at some point in their lives. However, most HPV infections do not lead to cervical cancer, and the body's immune system usually clears the infection on its own. Only a small percentage of women with persistent HPV infections will develop cervical cancer.

Symptoms of cervical cancer may not appear until the cancer has advanced. The most common symptom is abnormal vaginal bleeding, such as bleeding between periods, after sexual intercourse, or after menopause. Other symptoms may include pelvic pain or discomfort during sex, unusual vaginal discharge, or urinary symptoms.

Cervical cancer is usually diagnosed through a Pap test, which involves taking a sample of cells from the cervix and examining them under a microscope for abnormalities. If abnormal cells are found, a follow-up test called a colposcopy may be performed, which involves examining the cervix with a special magnifying device and taking a biopsy of any suspicious areas.

Treatment for cervical cancer depends on the stage of cancer and may include surgery, radiation therapy, chemotherapy, or a combination of these treatments. In the early stages, surgery is often the preferred option, while more advanced stages may require a combination of radiation and chemotherapy.

The best way to prevent cervical cancer is through regular cervical cancer screening, which includes regular Pap tests and HPV testing. The HPV vaccine is also highly effective in preventing the types of HPV that are most commonly associated with cervical cancer. Other measures that can reduce the risk of cervical cancer include practicing safe sex, quitting smoking, and maintaining a healthy immune system through a healthy diet and regular exercise.

Causes and Risk Factors

The main cause of cervical cancer is the human papillomavirus (HPV), a sexually transmitted infection that can cause abnormal changes in the cells of the cervix. However, not all women who are infected with HPV will develop cervical cancer, and other factors can increase the risk of developing the disease.

Here are some of the known risk factors for cervical cancer:

1. HPV infection: As mentioned, HPV is the primary cause of cervical cancer. Certain types of HPV are more strongly associated with cervical cancer than others, such as HPV types 16 and 18.
2. Age: Cervical cancer is most commonly diagnosed in women between the ages of 35 and 44. However, women of all ages can develop the disease.
3. Sexual activity: Sexually active Women are at a higher risk of developing cervical cancer than women who are not. This is because sexual activity increases the risk of HPV infection.

4. Multiple sexual partners: Women who have had multiple sexual partners or have had sex with someone who has had multiple partners are at a higher risk of developing cervical cancer.
5. Smoking: Women who smoke are more likely to develop cervical cancer than nonsmokers. This is because smoking can damage the DNA in cervical cells and weaken the immune system.
6. Weakened immune system: Women with weakened immune systems are at a higher risk of developing cervical cancer. This can be due to conditions such as HIV/AIDS or the use of immunosuppressive medications.
7. Family history: Women with a family history of cervical cancer are at a higher risk of developing the disease.
8. Birth control pills: Some studies have suggested that long-term use of birth control pills may increase the risk of cervical cancer.

It is important to note that having one or more risk factors does not necessarily mean that a woman will develop cervical cancer, and many women with no known risk factors still develop the disease. The best way to reduce the risk of cervical cancer is to undergo regular cervical cancer screening and practice safe sex.

Signs and Symptoms

In the early stages, cervical cancer may not cause any symptoms. However, as cancer grows, it may cause the following signs and symptoms:

1. Abnormal vaginal bleeding: This is the most common symptom of cervical cancer. It may include bleeding between periods, after sex, or after menopause.
2. Unusual vaginal discharge: Cervical cancer may cause a watery or bloody vaginal discharge that may have a foul odor.
3. Pelvic pain: Women with cervical cancer may experience pain or discomfort in the pelvic area, including during sex.
4. Pain during urination: As cancer grows, it may put pressure on the bladder, causing pain or discomfort during urination.
5. Leg swelling: In advanced stages of cervical cancer, cancer may spread to the lymph nodes in the pelvis or abdomen, causing swelling in the legs.

It is important to note that these symptoms can be caused by conditions other than cervical cancer, so it is important to talk to a healthcare provider if any of these symptoms occur.

Women should also undergo regular cervical cancer screening, which can detect abnormal changes in the cervix before symptoms develop.

Types of Cervical Cancer

There are two main types of cervical cancer:

1. Squamous cell carcinoma: This type of cervical cancer develops in the thin, flat cells that line the outer surface of the cervix.

2. Adenocarcinoma: This type of cervical cancer develops in the glandular cells that line the inner surface of the cervix.

Diagnosis and Staging

The diagnosis of cervical cancer typically involves several steps, including:

1. Pap test: This is a screening test that involves collecting cells from the cervix to be examined under a microscope. Abnormal cells can indicate the presence of cervical cancer.
2. HPV test: This test looks for the presence of the human papillomavirus (HPV) in cells from the cervix. HPV is a common cause of cervical cancer.
3. Biopsy: If abnormal cells are detected during a Pap test or HPV test, a biopsy may be performed. This involves removing a small sample of cervical tissue for examination under a microscope.
4. Imaging tests: Imaging tests such as X-rays, CT scans, MRI scans, or PET scans may be done to determine if cancer has spread to other parts of the body.
5. Colposcopy: This is a visual examination of the cervix using a special instrument called a colposcopy. It is usually performed if abnormal cells are detected on a Pap smear or HPV test.

6. Imaging tests: Imaging tests such as X-rays, CT scans, or MRI scans may be used to determine the extent of cancer and whether it has spread to other parts of the body.

It's important to note that the specific tests used may vary depending on the individual patient's situation and the recommendations of their healthcare provider.

The staging of cervical cancer is based on the results of diagnostic tests and determines the extent of the cancer. The most commonly used staging system for cervical cancer is the FIGO staging system, which includes the following stages:

Stage 0: Abnormal cells are found on the surface of the cervix, but cancer has not spread beyond this layer.

Stage I: The cancer is present only in the cervix.

Stage II: Cancer has spread beyond the cervix, but not to the pelvic wall or the lower third of the vagina.

Stage III: Cancer has spread to the pelvic wall or the lower third of the vagina.

Stage IV: Cancer has spread to other parts of the body, such as the bladder, rectum, or distant organs.

The staging of cervical cancer is important because it helps determine the most appropriate treatment options and provides information about the expected outcome of the disease.

Once the staging process is complete, the healthcare provider will discuss the results with the patient and recommend a treatment plan based on the stage of cancer and other factors such as the patient's age and overall health. The treatment plan may include surgery, radiation therapy, chemotherapy, or a combination of these treatments. The healthcare provider will also discuss the possible side effects of the treatment and the expected outcome. It's important to ask questions and discuss any concerns with the healthcare provider to fully understand the staging process and what to expect during treatment.

Screening Tests in Cervical Cancer

Screening tests for cervical cancer aim to detect the presence of pre-cancerous or cancerous cells in the cervix before symptoms appear. The most common screening tests for cervical cancer include:

1. Pap test (Pap smear): This test involves collecting cells from the cervix and examining them under a microscope to detect any abnormal cells. It is recommended for women starting at age 21 and repeating every 3 years for women aged 21-29. Women aged 30-65 may do a Pap test every 5 years or a combination of Pap test and HPV test every 5 years.
2. HPV test: This test checks for the presence of high-risk strains of the human papillomavirus (HPV), which is the primary cause of cervical cancer. It is recommended for women aged 30-65 and may be used in combination with a Pap test.
3. Visual Inspection with Acetic Acid (VIA): This involves applying a solution of acetic acid to the cervix and inspecting it visually for any abnormal areas. This test is commonly used in low-resource settings.

4. Visual Inspection with Lugol's Iodine (VILI): This test involves applying a solution of Lugol's iodine to the cervix and inspecting it visually for any abnormal areas. This test is also used in low-resource settings.

Women need to discuss with their healthcare provider which screening test is appropriate for them based on their age, medical history, and risk factors. Regular screening can help detect cervical cancer early when it is most treatable.

Treatment Options

Treatment options for cervical cancer depend on several factors, including the stage of cancer, the patient's age and overall health, and the patient's personal preferences. Some common treatment options for cervical cancer include:

1. Surgery: Surgery is often the first treatment option for early-stage cervical cancer. It involves removing the cancerous tissue and may involve removing the uterus, cervix, and surrounding tissue.
2. Radiation therapy: Radiation therapy uses high-energy X-rays or other types of radiation to kill cancer cells. It is often used in combination with other treatments, such as surgery or chemotherapy.
3. Chemotherapy: Chemotherapy involves the use of drugs to kill cancer cells. It is often used in combination with other treatments, such as surgery or radiation therapy.
4. Targeted therapy: Targeted therapy uses drugs to target specific proteins or other molecules that are involved in the growth and spread of cancer cells.

5. Immunotherapy: Immunotherapy uses drugs to stimulate the immune system to attack cancer cells.
6. Palliative care: Palliative care focuses on providing relief from symptoms and improving the quality of life for patients with advanced cervical cancer.

The choice of treatment will depend on the individual patient's circumstances, and a multidisciplinary team including a gynecologic oncologist, radiation oncologist, medical oncologist, and other specialists will work together to develop a personalized treatment plan.

Surgery treatment

Surgery is one of the main treatments for cervical cancer. The type of surgery recommended depends on the stage of cancer and other factors. The following are the common surgical procedures used to treat cervical cancer:

Radical hysterectomy: This surgery involves removing the uterus, cervix, upper part of the vagina, and the supporting tissues around these organs. This is usually recommended for early-stage cervical cancer.

Radical trachelectomy: This surgery involves removing the cervix and the upper part of the vagina while preserving the uterus. This is an option for women who want to preserve their fertility.

Pelvic exenterating: This is a major surgery that involves removing the uterus, cervix, vagina, ovaries, fallopian tubes, bladder, and rectum. This surgery is usually recommended for advanced cervical cancer that has spread to nearby organs.

In addition to these surgeries, lymph nodes in the pelvis may also be removed to check for the spread of cancer. Surgery may be done alone or in combination with other treatments such as radiation therapy and chemotherapy.

It's important to discuss the benefits and risks of surgery with your doctor, as well as any potential side effects and long-term effects on fertility and sexual function. Your doctor will help you make an informed decision about the best treatment plan for you.

Radiation therapy

Radiation therapy is a common treatment option for cervical cancer. It uses high-energy X-rays or other types of radiation to kill cancer cells and shrink tumors.

Radiation therapy may be used alone or in combination with other treatments, such as surgery and chemotherapy.

There are two main types of radiation therapy for cervical cancer: external beam radiation therapy and brachytherapy.

External beam radiation therapy: This type of radiation therapy uses a machine outside the body to deliver radiation to cancer. The radiation is focused on the pelvis, where the cervix and surrounding tissue are located. External beam radiation therapy is typically given five days a week for several weeks.

Brachytherapy: Brachytherapy involves placing a radioactive source, such as a small tube, inside the vagina or cervix for a short period. The radiation is delivered directly to the cancer and surrounding tissue. Brachytherapy may be given alone or in combination with external beam radiation therapy.

Radiation therapy can have side effects, including fatigue, skin irritation, and gastrointestinal problems. However, most side effects are temporary and can be managed with medication or lifestyle changes. Patients should discuss the potential side effects of radiation therapy with their healthcare team and follow their recommendations for managing them.

Overall, radiation therapy can be an effective treatment option for cervical cancer, particularly when used in combination with other treatments. The choice of radiation therapy will depend on the stage of cancer, the location of the tumor, and the patient's overall health.

Chemotherapy treatment

Chemotherapy is a cancer treatment that uses drugs to kill cancer cells. It is often used in combination with other treatments, such as surgery and radiation therapy, for cervical cancer.

Chemotherapy drugs work by targeting rapidly dividing cells, including cancer cells. The drugs are given either orally or through a vein, and travel through the bloodstream to reach cancer cells throughout the body.

Chemotherapy can be given before or after surgery, or along with radiation therapy. When given before surgery, it is called neoadjuvant chemotherapy. This type of chemotherapy can help shrink the tumor and make it easier to remove during surgery. When given after surgery, it is called adjuvant chemotherapy. This type of chemotherapy can help kill any remaining cancer cells after surgery and reduce the risk of cancer coming back.

Chemotherapy can have side effects, including nausea, vomiting, hair loss, fatigue, and an increased risk of infection. However, many side effects can be managed with medication or lifestyle changes.

Overall, chemotherapy can be an effective treatment option for cervical cancer, particularly when used in combination with other treatments. The choice of chemotherapy will depend on the stage of cancer, the patient's overall health, and other factors. Patients should discuss the potential benefits and side effects of chemotherapy with their healthcare team and follow their recommendations for managing them.

Targeted therapy

Targeted therapy is a type of cancer treatment that uses drugs to target specific molecules or proteins that are involved in the growth and spread of cancer cells. These drugs work by blocking the signals that cancer cells use to grow and divide.

In cervical cancer, targeted therapy is often used in combination with chemotherapy. One targeted therapy drug that has been approved for the treatment of cervical cancer is bevacizumab, which works by blocking the growth of blood vessels that supply the tumor with nutrients and oxygen.

Targeted therapy is usually given intravenously, and the treatment schedule depends on the specific drug being used. It is often used in advanced or recurrent cervical cancer, but it may also be used in combination with other treatments for earlier stages of the disease.

Targeted therapy can have side effects, including high blood pressure, fatigue, gastrointestinal problems, and an increased risk of bleeding. However, many side effects can be managed with medication or lifestyle changes.

Overall, targeted therapy can be an effective treatment option for cervical cancer, particularly when used in combination with other treatments. The choice of targeted therapy will depend on the stage of cancer, the patient's overall health, and other factors. Patients should discuss the potential benefits and side effects of targeted therapy with their healthcare team and follow their recommendations for managing them.

Immunotherapy

Immunotherapy is a type of cancer treatment that uses the body's immune system to fight cancer. In cervical cancer, immunotherapy is usually used in advanced or recurrent diseases.

There are different types of immunotherapy, but the most commonly used type for cervical cancer is checkpoint inhibitors. These drugs work by blocking certain proteins in cancer cells that can inhibit the immune system's ability to attack them.

One checkpoint inhibitor drug that has been approved for the treatment of cervical cancer is pembrolizumab. It is usually given intravenously every three weeks.

Immunotherapy can have side effects, including fatigue, skin rash, diarrhea, and an increased risk of infection. However, many side effects can be managed with medication or lifestyle changes.

Overall, immunotherapy can be an effective treatment option for cervical cancer, particularly when used in combination with other treatments. The choice of immunotherapy will depend on the stage of cancer, the patient's overall health, and other factors. Patients should discuss the potential benefits and side effects of immunotherapy with their healthcare team and follow their recommendations for managing them.

Coping With the Side Effects of Treatment

Coping with the side effects of cervical cancer treatment can be challenging, but some strategies can help. Here are some tips for managing common side effects:

Fatigue: Get plenty of rest and try to conserve energy by prioritizing tasks and delegating responsibilities. Light exercises such as walking or yoga may also help to boost energy levels.

Nausea and vomiting: Eat small, frequent meals and avoid spicy, greasy, or high-fat foods. Drinking plenty of fluids and avoiding strong odors may also help to reduce nausea.

Hair loss: Consider wearing a wig or other head covering, or simply embrace your new look. Some people find it helpful to involve loved ones in the process, such as having a "shaving party" before the hair falls out.

Skin changes: Use gentle skincare products and avoid exposure to the sun or other sources of heat such as hot water or heating pads. Moisturizing regularly and wearing loose-fitting clothing may also help to soothe the skin.

Changes in appetite: Eat small, frequent meals and

try to incorporate nutrient-rich foods such as fruits, vegetables, and whole grains. Consult with a registered dietitian for personalized nutrition advice.

Emotional distress: It's normal to experience a range of emotions during treatment, such as anxiety, depression, or fear. Consider seeking support from a therapist or counselor, joining a support group, or confiding in a trusted friend or family member.

It's important to communicate with your healthcare provider about any side effects you may be experiencing, as they may be able to offer additional strategies or adjust your treatment plan as needed. With time and support, many people can manage the side effects of cervical cancer treatment and maintain a good quality of life.

Physical side effects and how to manage them

Fatigue: Feeling extremely tired, even after rest or sleep. This is a common side effect of cervical cancer and its treatment.

How to manage fatigue: Get plenty of rest and sleep, eat a healthy diet, and exercise when possible. Ask for help with household chores and other tasks. Talk to your healthcare provider about medications or other interventions that may help.

Nausea and vomiting: Some women experience nausea and vomiting during cervical cancer treatment.

How to manage nausea and vomiting: Try eating small, frequent meals throughout the day, and avoid fatty or spicy foods. Drink plenty of fluids, and ask your healthcare provider about anti-nausea medications.

Pain: Pain in the pelvic area or lower back may occur during cervical cancer treatment.

How to manage pain: Talk to your healthcare provider about pain management options, including over-the-counter or prescription pain relievers, physical therapy, or complementary therapies like acupuncture or massage.

Bowel and bladder problems: Treatment for cervical cancer can cause bowel and bladder problems, including diarrhea, constipation, and urinary incontinence.

How to manage bowel and bladder problems: Eat a healthy diet with plenty of fiber to help regulate bowel movements. Drink plenty of fluids to help flush out your urinary system, and practice Kegel exercises to help strengthen your pelvic muscles.

Sexual side effects: Women with cervical cancer may experience changes in their sexual function, including pain during intercourse or vaginal dryness.

How to manage sexual side effects: Talk to your healthcare provider about options for managing sexual side effects, including vaginal lubricants or hormone replacement therapy. Consider counseling or support groups to help address any emotional or relationship issues related to sexual changes.

Lymphedema: Lymphedema is swelling in the arms or legs that can occur after surgery or radiation for cervical cancer.

How to manage lymphedema: Wear compression garments or sleeves to help reduce swelling. Exercise regularly, but avoid activities that put too much strain on the affected limb. Practice good skin care, including keeping the affected limb clean and moisturized.

It's important to remember that each person's experience with cervical cancer and its treatment is unique, and not everyone will experience all of these side effects. Your healthcare provider can work with you to develop a personalized plan for managing any physical side effects you may experience.

Emotional and mental health considerations

Here are some key factors to consider:

Coping with a cancer diagnosis: A cancer diagnosis can be overwhelming and emotionally challenging. It is important to address the emotional impact of a diagnosis and provide guidance on how to cope with the emotional rollercoaster that comes with it.

Managing stress and anxiety: Cancer treatment can be stressful and anxiety-provoking. It is important to provide strategies for managing stress and anxiety, such as mindfulness, meditation, or exercise.

Addressing fears and concerns: Survivors of cervical cancer may have fears and concerns about their health, future fertility, or intimate relationships. It is important to provide resources and support for addressing these concerns.

Dealing with physical changes: Survivors of cervical cancer may experience physical changes, such as scarring, infertility, or sexual dysfunction. It is important to address these changes and provide resources for managing them.

Maintaining social support: Cancer survivors may feel isolated or alone. It is important to guide on maintaining social support and building a support network of family, friends, and healthcare professionals.

Addressing survivorship issues: Survivors of cervical cancer may face long-term physical and emotional challenges. It is important to address survivorship issues, such as ongoing medical follow-up, managing chronic pain, and maintaining emotional and mental well-being.

Overall, addressing emotional and mental health considerations is an important aspect of writing a book on surviving cervical cancer. By addressing coping strategies, stress management, fears and concerns, physical changes, social support, and survivorship issues, the book can provide comprehensive guidance for survivors and help them thrive in their daily lives.

Support systems and resources

There are several support systems and resources available for those who have been diagnosed with cervical cancer or for those who are looking to learn more about the condition. Here are a few resources to consider:

Cancer Support Community: This is a global nonprofit organization that provides support and resources for cancer patients and its 24/7 helpline, online support groups, and a database of local resources.

National Cervical Cancer Coalition: This organization is dedicated to raising awareness about cervical cancer and providing support for those affected by the disease. They offer resources such as support groups, educational materials, and a helpline.

Cervivor: This is a nonprofit organization that provides support and advocacy for cervical cancer survivors. They offer a variety of resources, including a mentorship program, online support groups, and educational materials.

The Women's Cancer Network: This organization provides information and support for women with all types of cancer, including cervical cancer. They offer resources such as online support groups, educational materials, and a helpline.

In addition to these organizations, there may be local support groups and resources available in your area. Your doctor or healthcare provider may be able to provide you with information about these resources.

It's also worth checking with your insurance provider to see if they offer any support programs for cancer patients.

Living after Cervical Cancer

Living after cervical cancer can be challenging, but there are many things you can do to improve your quality of life and regain your sense of well-being. Here are some tips that may help:

Stay physically active: Regular exercise can help improve your mood, boost your energy levels, and reduce your risk of other health problems. Talk to your doctor about what type and level of exercise is safe for you.

Eat a healthy diet: A healthy diet that's rich in fruits, vegetables, whole grains, and lean proteins can help you maintain your energy levels and reduce your risk of other health problems.

Connect with others: Talking to others who have gone through a similar experience can be very helpful. Joining a support group or connecting with others online can help you feel less alone and provide you with valuable support and information.

Practice self-care: Make time for activities that you enjoy, such as reading, meditating, or spending time with friends and family.

Taking care of yourself can help reduce stress and improve your overall sense of well-being.

Attend follow-up appointments: It's important to attend all your follow-up appointments with your doctor, even if you're feeling well. These appointments can help you detect any potential problems early and help you stay healthy.

Remember, it's normal to experience a wide range of emotions after a cancer diagnosis. It's important to give yourself time to process your feelings and seek help if you need it. With time, patience, and the right support, you can move forward and enjoy a fulfilling life after cervical cancer.

Follow-up care

If you or someone you know has survived cervical cancer, it is important to receive proper follow-up care to ensure that the cancer has not returned and to address any other health concerns related to the cancer treatment. Here are some important steps to take:

Regular follow-up appointments with your healthcare provider: Your healthcare provider will monitor your health and conduct regular pelvic exams, Pap tests, and other tests as needed to check for signs of cancer recurrence.

Discuss your fertility options: If you are of childbearing age and wish to have children, talk to your healthcare provider about your options for preserving your fertility before undergoing cancer treatment.

Address any side effects of treatment: Cancer treatment can have long-term effects on your body, including issues with fertility, sexual function, and urinary or bowel function. Talk to your healthcare provider about any ongoing symptoms or side effects you may be experiencing and discuss potential treatments or therapies to address them.

Maintain a healthy lifestyle: Eating a healthy diet, getting regular exercise, and avoiding smoking and excessive alcohol consumption can help reduce your risk of cancer recurrence and improve your overall health and well-being.

Seek support: Surviving cancer can be a challenging experience, and it is important to seek emotional support from loved ones, support groups, or mental health professionals to help you cope with any ongoing physical or emotional challenges.

Remember to always follow your healthcare provider's recommendations for follow-up care and to stay vigilant about your health and well-being after surviving cervical cancer.

Lifestyle Changes to Reduce the Risk of Recurrence

Lifestyle changes can play an important role in reducing the risk of recurrence of cervical cancer. Here are some lifestyle changes you may want to consider:

Stop smoking: Smoking can increase the risk of cervical cancer recurrence. Encourage readers who smoke to quit smoking and provide resources to help them quit.

Exercise regularly: Regular exercise can help reduce the risk of recurrence and improve overall health. Encourage readers to aim for at least 30 minutes of moderate exercise most days of the week.

Eat a healthy diet: Eating a diet that is rich in fruits, vegetables, whole grains, lean protein, and healthy fats can help improve overall health and reduce the risk of cancer recurrence. Encourage readers to avoid processed foods, sugary drinks, and excessive amounts of red meat.

Manage stress: Stress can weaken the immune system and increase inflammation in the body, both of which can increase the risk of cancer recurrence.

Encourage readers to find healthy ways to manage stress, such as through meditation, yoga, or talking with a therapist.

Get regular check-ups: Encourage readers to see their doctor regularly for check-ups and follow-up tests, as recommended by their healthcare provider. This can help detect any potential recurrence early and improve outcomes.

Avoid risky behaviors: Encourage readers to avoid risky behaviors, such as having unprotected sex or using drugs that can increase the risk of HPV infection or weaken the immune system.

By incorporating these lifestyle changes, you can help reduce the risk of recurrence of cervical cancer and improve your overall health and well-being.

Emotional Healing and Finding a New Normal

Emotional healing and finding a new normal after cervical cancer treatment is an important part of the recovery process. Here are some tips that may help you:

Allow yourself to grieve: It's natural to feel a range of emotions after a cancer diagnosis and treatment, including sadness, anger, and fear. Encourage your readers to allow themselves to feel these emotions and seek support from loved ones or a mental health professional if needed.

Take things one day at a time: Recovery after cancer treatment can be overwhelming, so encourage readers to focus on taking things one day at a time. Setting small goals can help them feel a sense of accomplishment and progress.

Seek support: Encourage readers to seek support from others who have gone through similar experiences, such as a support group or an online community. Connecting with others who understand what they are going through can help reduce feelings of isolation and provide a sense of belonging.

Practice self-care: Encourage readers to prioritize self-care activities that promote relaxation and well-being, such as getting enough sleep, practicing mindfulness or meditation, and engaging in physical activity they enjoy.

Set boundaries: Encourage readers to set boundaries with others if they are feeling overwhelmed or need time to focus on their healing. This can include saying no to commitments that are too demanding or setting limits on how much they share about their experiences with others.

Celebrate milestones: Encourage readers to celebrate milestones in their recovery, such as finishing treatment, reaching a physical or emotional goal, or returning to work or other activities. Celebrating these achievements can help boost their confidence and sense of accomplishment.

By focusing on emotional healing and finding a new normal after cervical cancer treatment, you can work towards a fulfilling and healthy future.

Conclusion

Cervical cancer can be a challenging diagnosis, but there are many treatment options available, including surgery, radiation therapy, chemotherapy, targeted therapy, and immunotherapy. The choice of treatment will depend on the stage of cancer, the patient's overall health, and other factors. Patients need to work closely with their healthcare team to determine the best treatment plan for their individual needs.

In addition to medical treatment, there are many resources and support options available for cervical cancer patients, including national and local organizations, online support groups, and local cancer centers and hospitals. These resources can provide valuable information, support, and hope for patients and their families throughout their cancer journey.

Cervical cancer patients need to know that they are not alone and that there are many people and organizations available to support them through their cancer diagnosis, treatment, and recovery.

Looking Ahead and Staying Positive

Looking ahead and staying positive can be important aspects of the cervical cancer journey. Here are some tips for staying positive:

1. Focus on what you can control: While a cancer diagnosis can be overwhelming, focusing on what you can control can help you feel more empowered. This may include making healthy lifestyle choices, staying informed about your treatment options, and surrounding yourself with supportive people.

2. Practice self-care: Taking care of yourself can help improve your overall well-being and help you feel more positive. This may include getting enough sleep, eating a healthy diet, and engaging in activities that bring you joy and relaxation.

3. Seek support: Surrounding yourself with supportive people, such as family, friends, and support groups, can help you feel more optimistic. Talking to others who have gone through similar experiences can also help you feel less alone.

4. Stay informed: Educating yourself about your condition and treatment options can help you feel more in control and reduce anxiety.

However, be sure to get information from reputable sources, such as your healthcare team or national cancer organizations.

5. Set realistic goals: Setting small, achievable goals can help you feel more accomplished and positive. These goals may include exercising a few times a week, learning a new skill, or spending more time with loved ones.

Remember, staying positive doesn't mean ignoring the challenges of the cancer journey. It is okay to feel a range of emotions, including fear, sadness, and anger. However, by focusing on what you can control, practicing self-care, seeking support, staying informed, and setting realistic goals, you can stay positive and hopeful for the future.